Content:-

1. What is Yoga

Yoga is a mind and body practice with a 5,000-year history in ancient Indian philosophy. The practice entails low-impact physical activity, postures (called *asanas*), breathing techniques (*pranayama*), relaxation, and meditation. Most people are familiar with the physical poses or yoga positions but don't know that yoga involves so much more.

In more recent years, it has become popular as a form of physical exercise based upon poses that promote improved control of the mind and body and enhance well-being.There are several different types of yoga and many disciplines within the practice

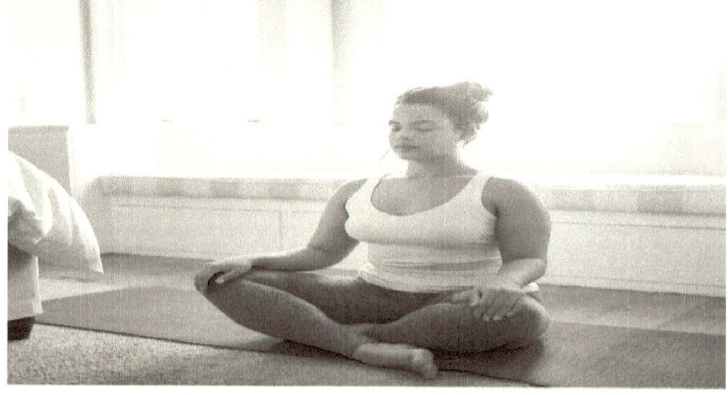

2. Why Yoga is Compulsory

If you want to remain in good health, these all are compulsory. It will increase your health life. Many doctors recommend you to do yoga, exercise and meditation to remain in good health. You should have to extract 30 min - 60 min daily for this. If you regularly do this, you will never face any health issue.

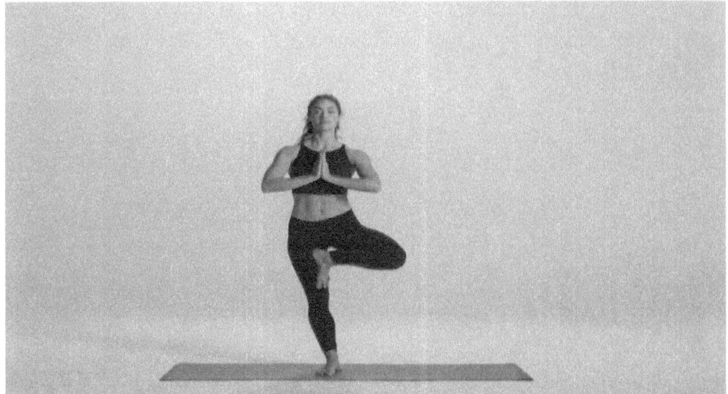

3. Benefits of Yoga

Following are the benefits of yoga, exercise and meditation.

- **Supports your connective tissue**

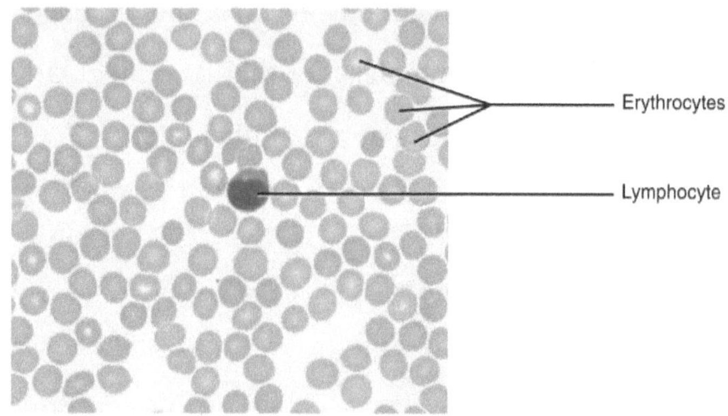

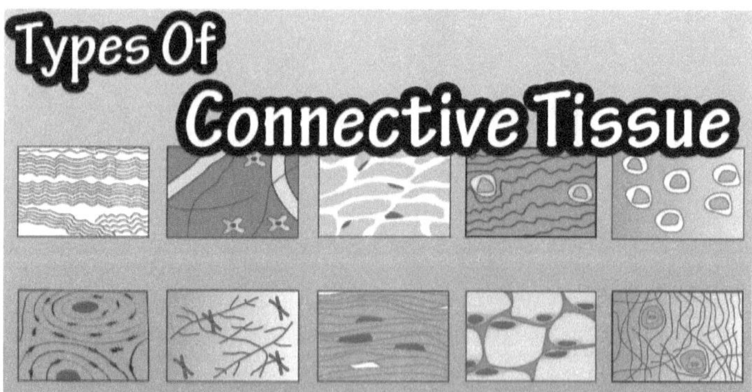

- **Encourages self care**

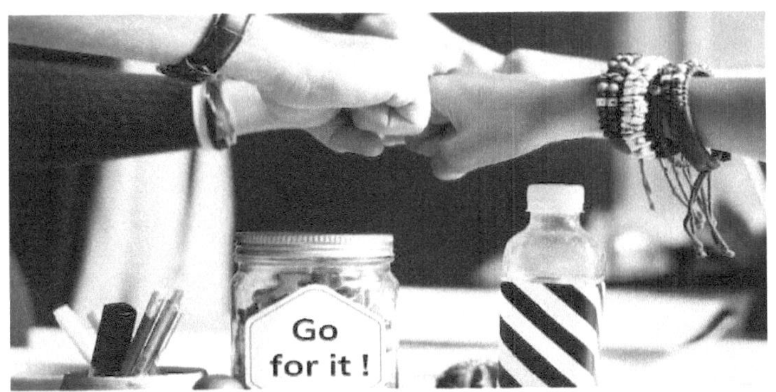

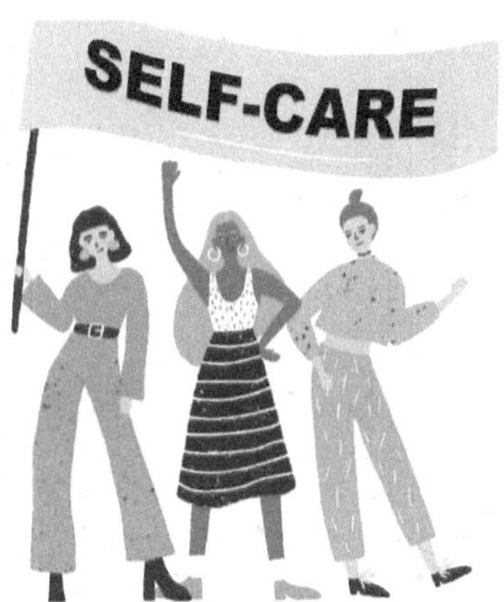

-    **Keeps allergies and viruses at bay**

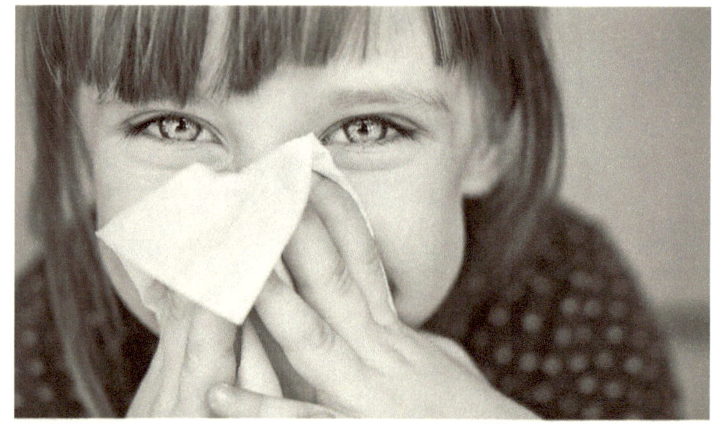

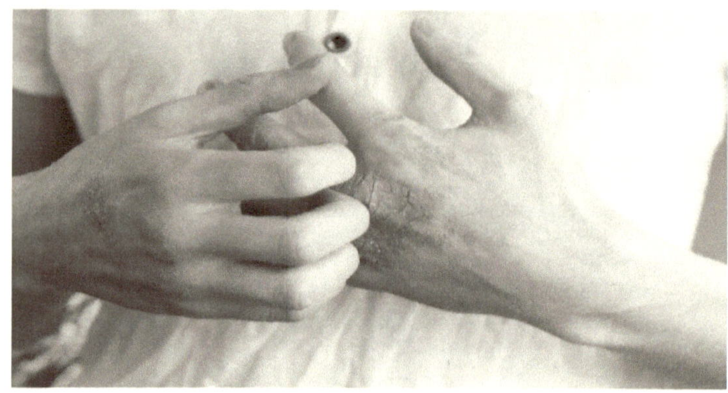

- **Helps keep you drug free**

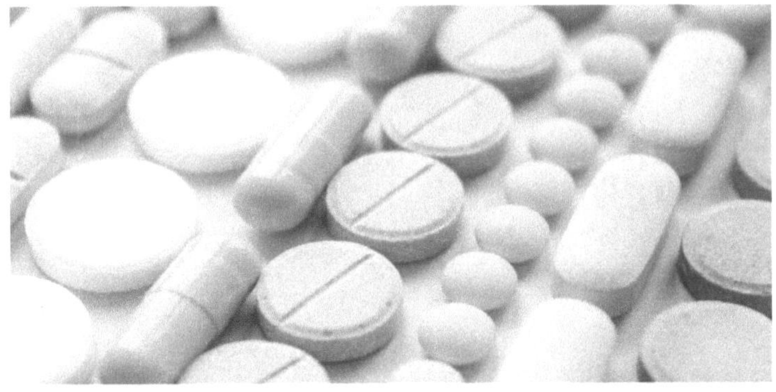

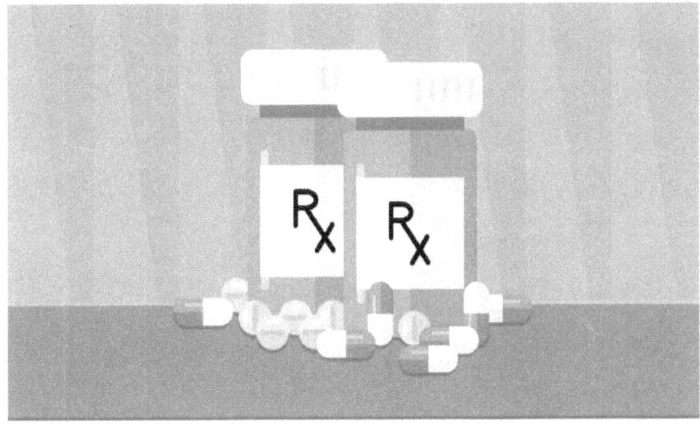

- **Gives you inner strength**

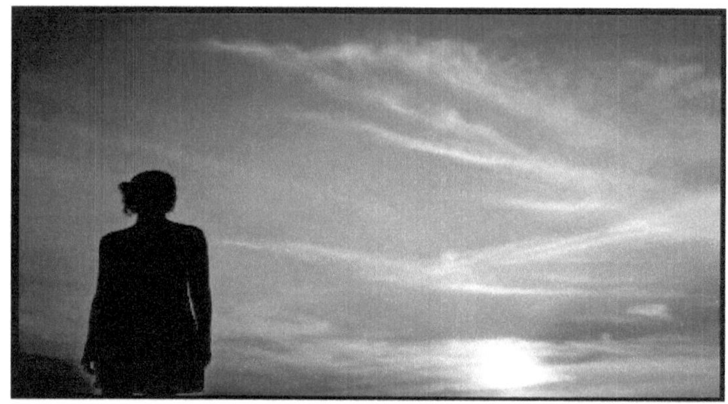

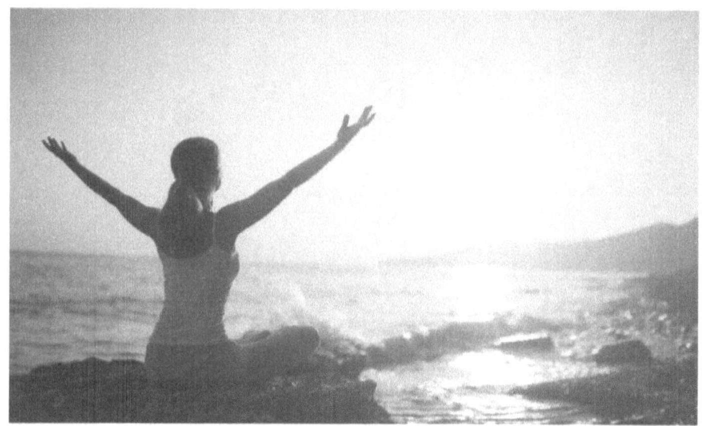

- **Eases your pain**

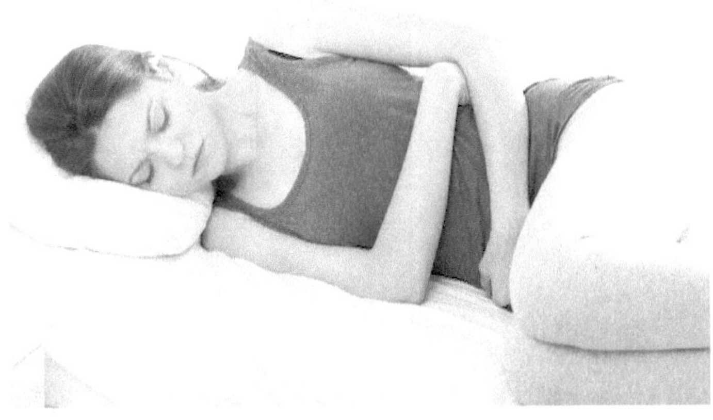

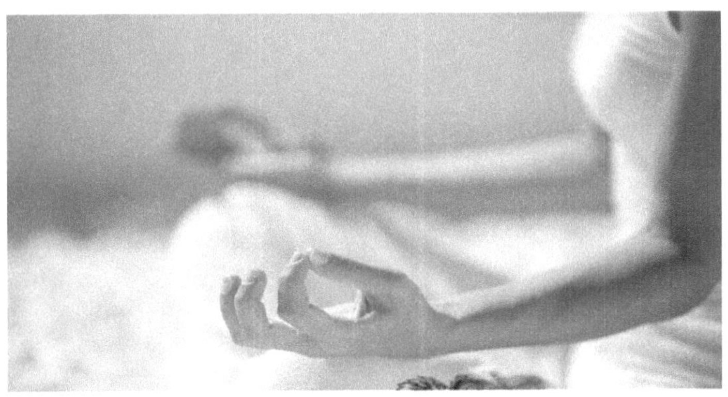

- **Increases your self-esteem**

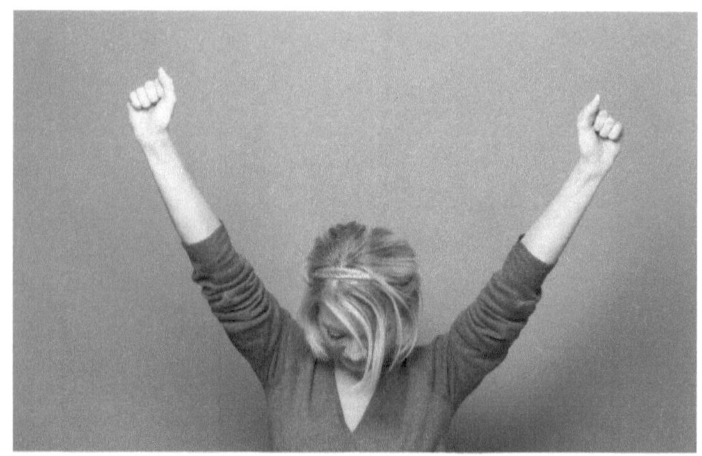

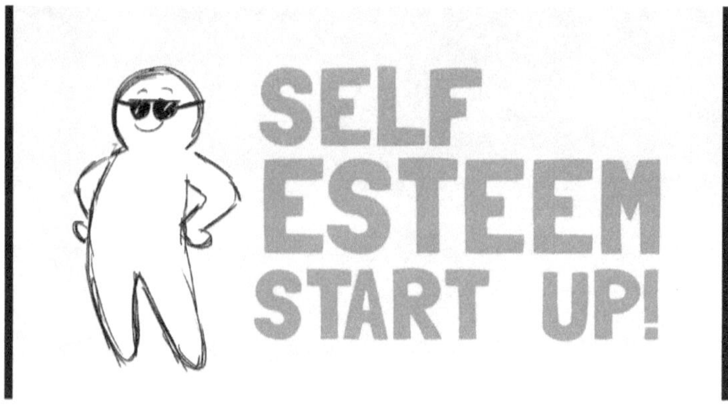

- **Gives you peace of mind**

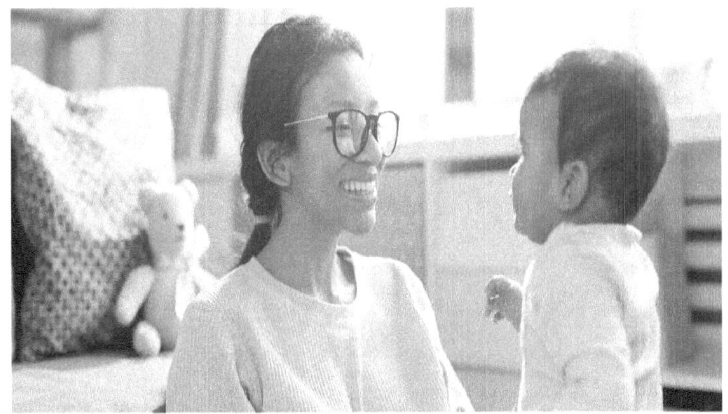

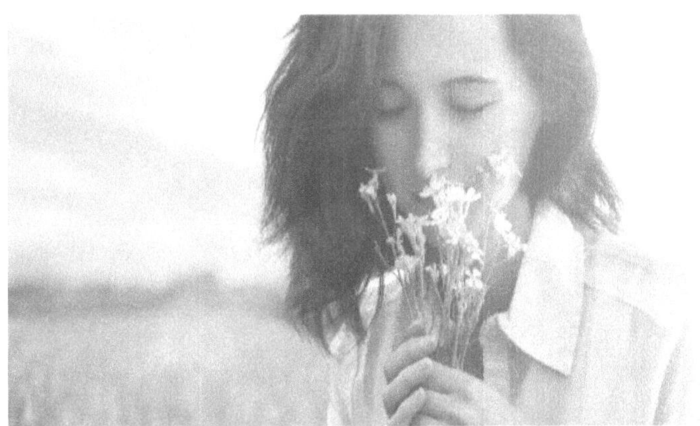

- **Prevents IBS and other digestive problems**

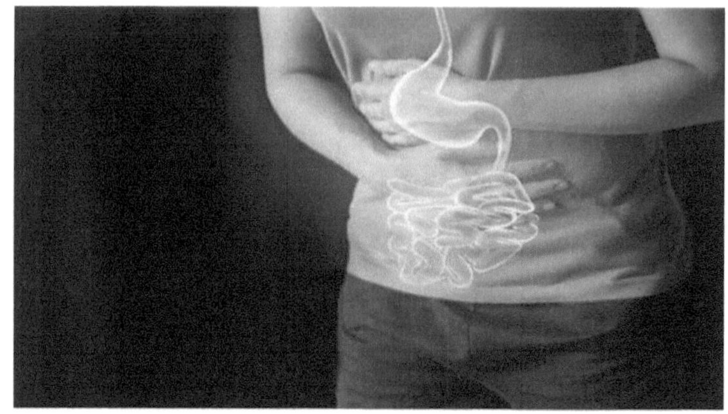

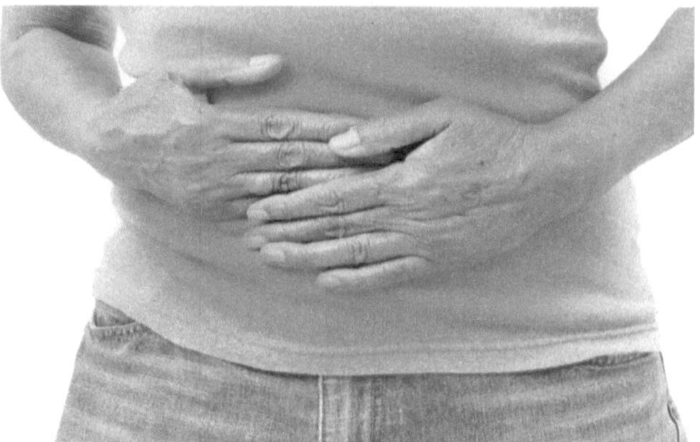

- **Gives your lungs room to breathe**

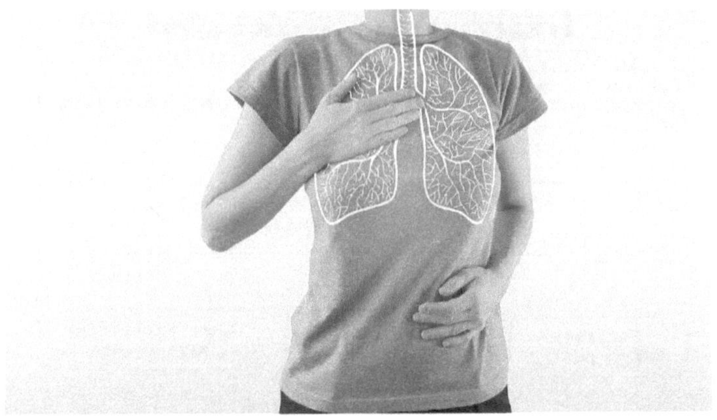

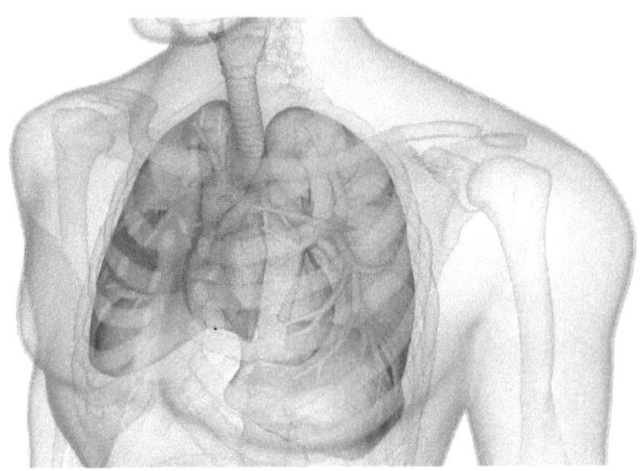

- **Boosts your immune system functionality**

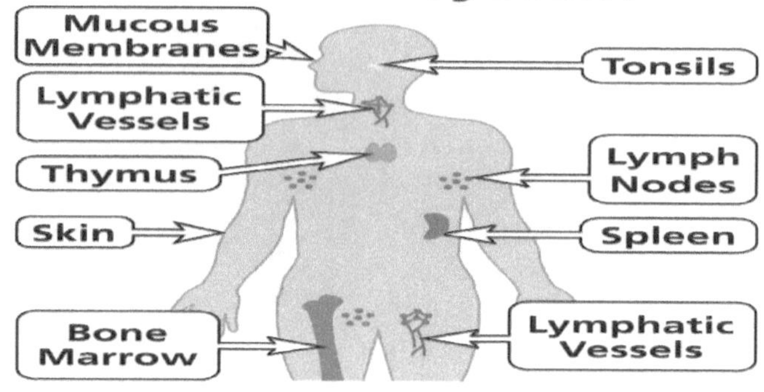

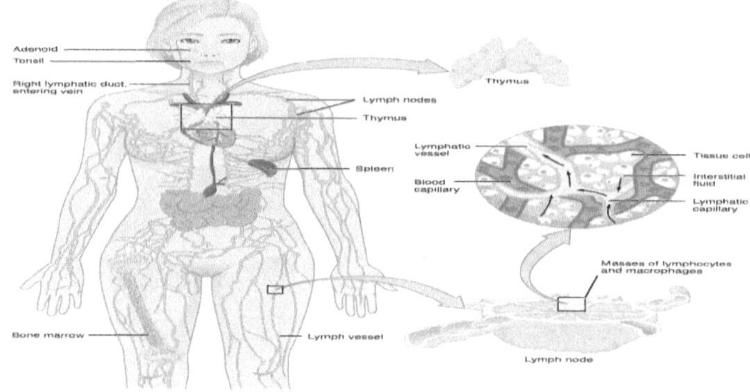

- **Helps you sleep deeper**

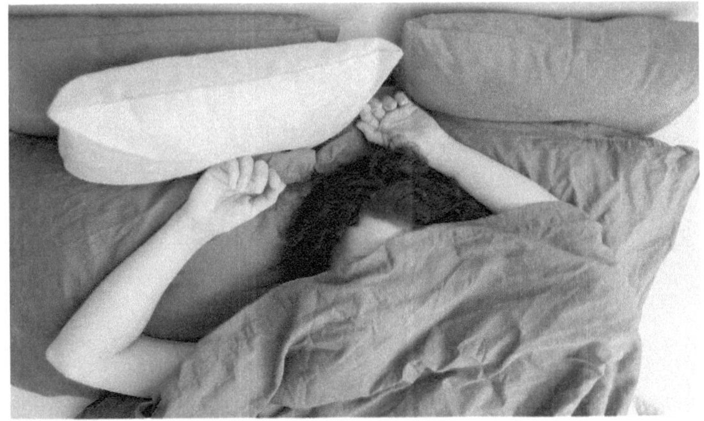

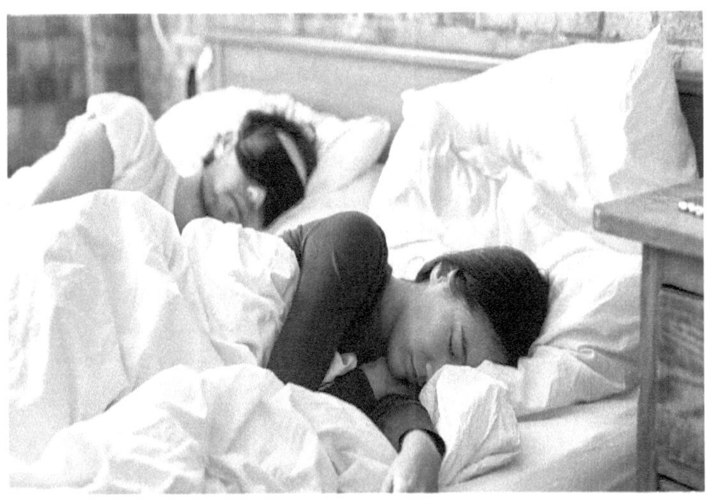

-     **Releases tension in your limbs**

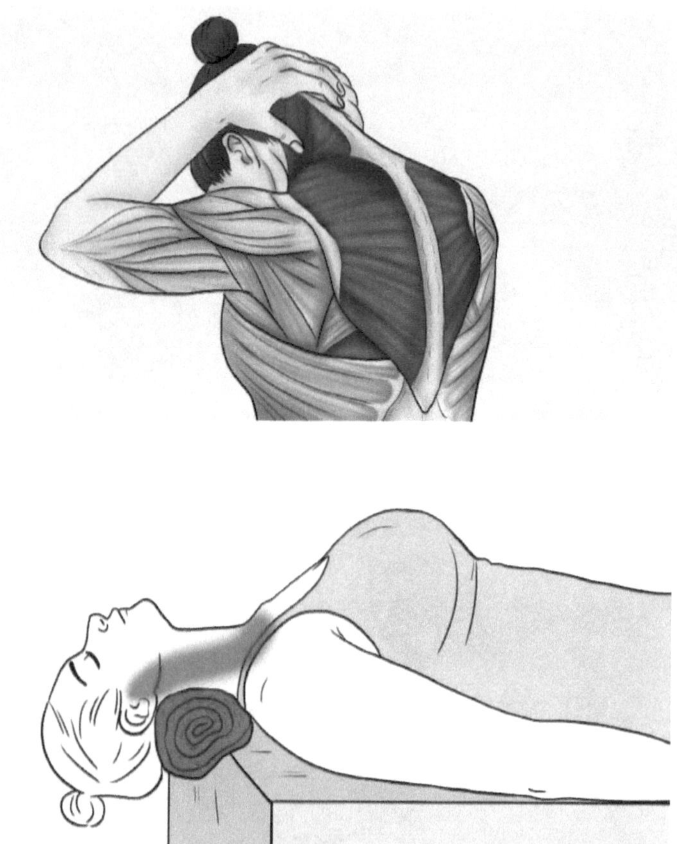

- **Maintains your nervous system**

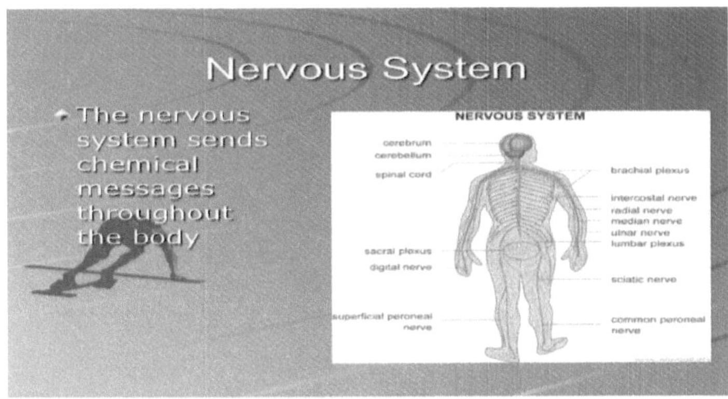

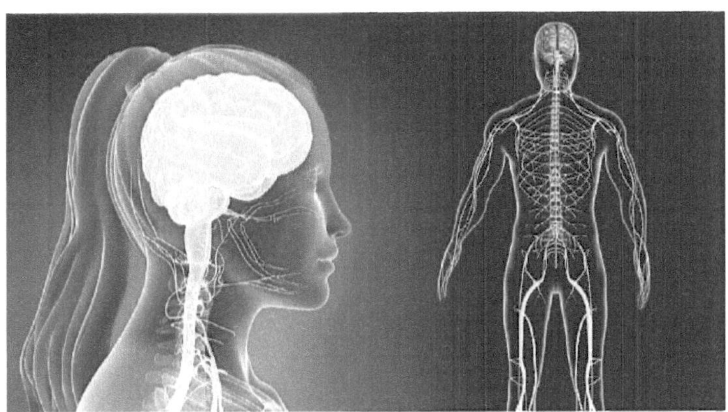

- **Improves your balance**

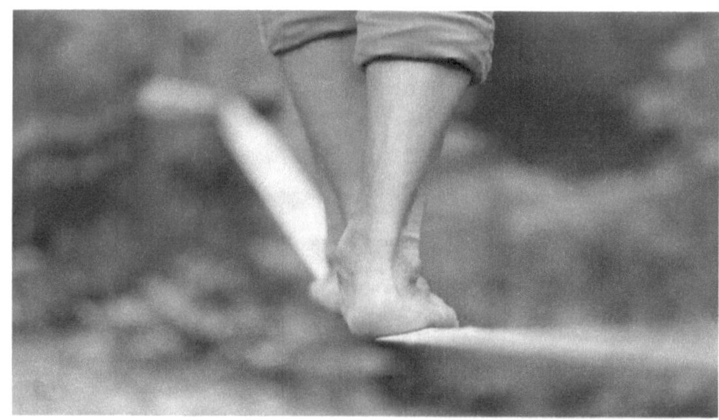

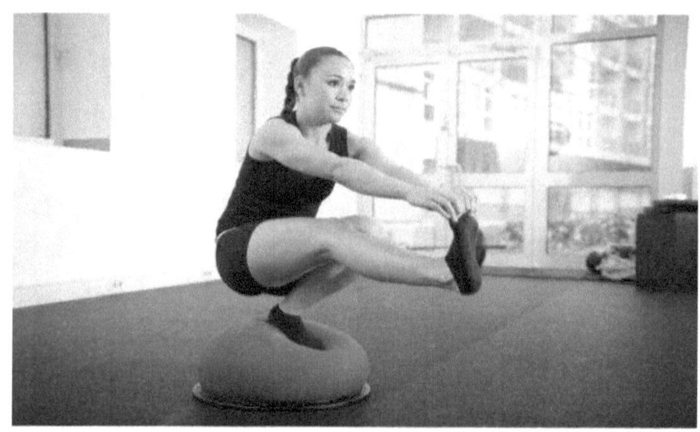

- **Relaxes your system**

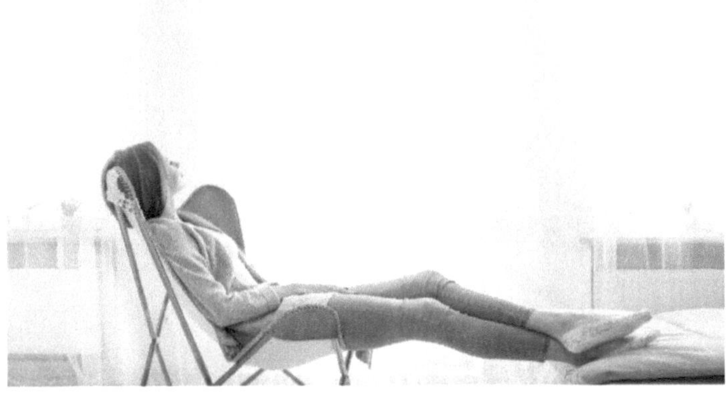

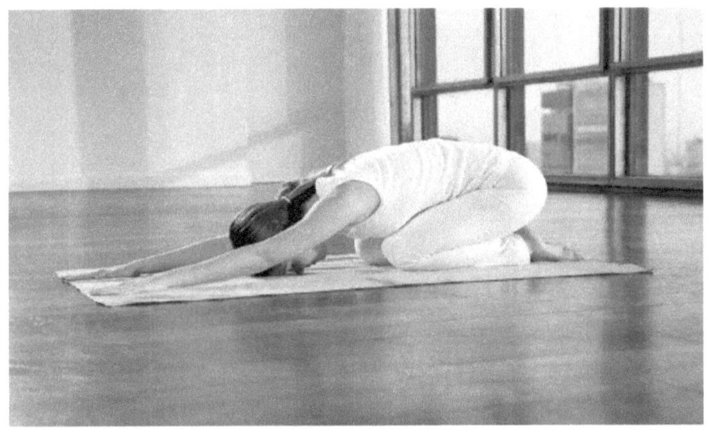

- **Helps you focus**

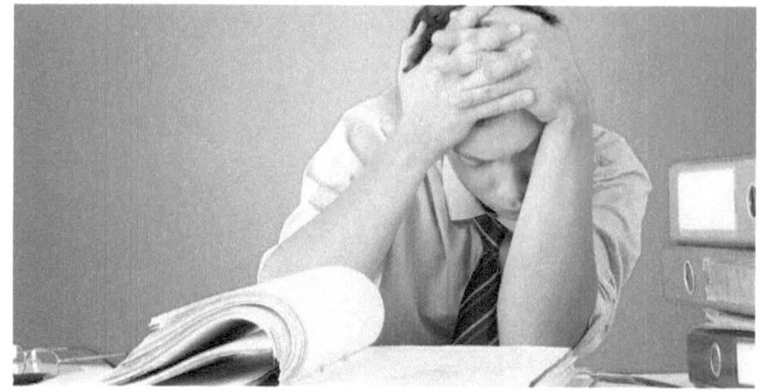

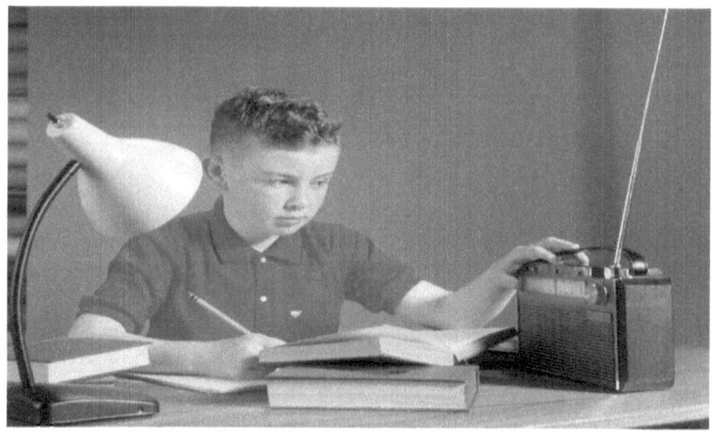

-    **Lowers blood sugar**

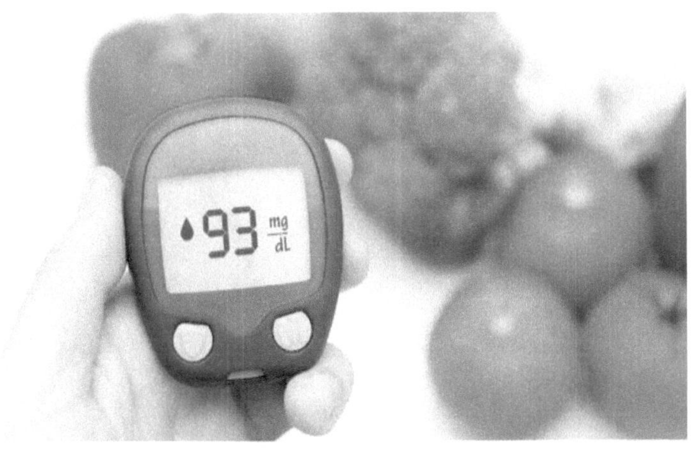

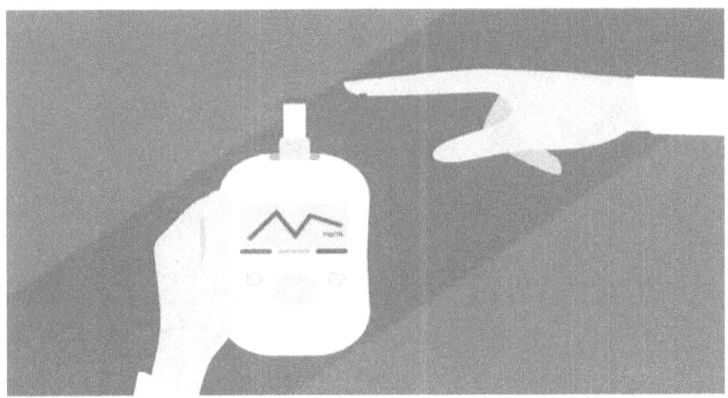

- **Founds a healthy lifestyle**

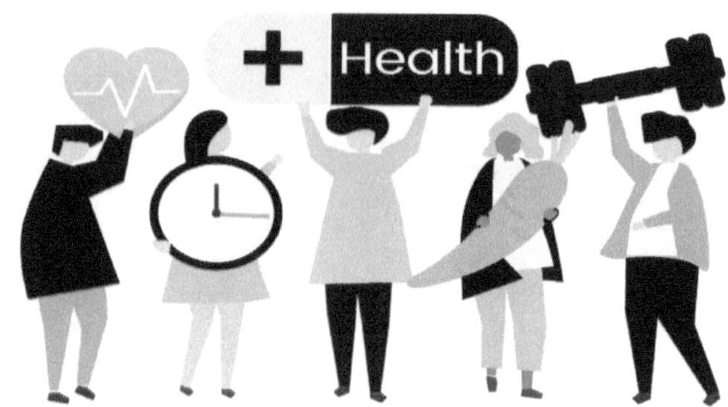

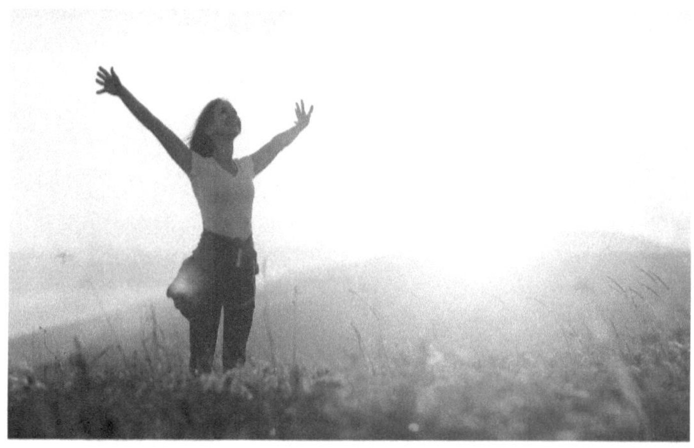

- **Makes you happier**

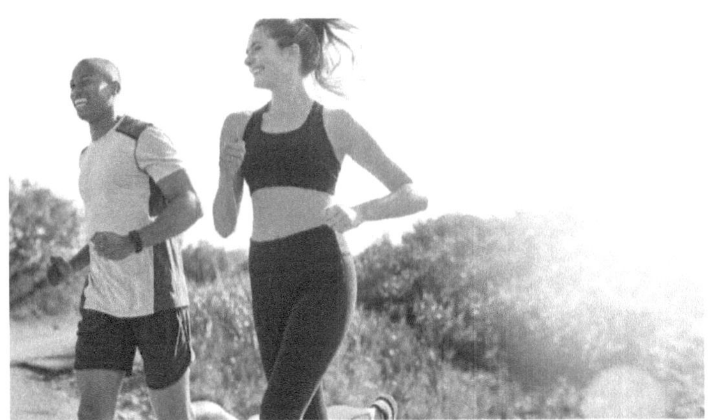

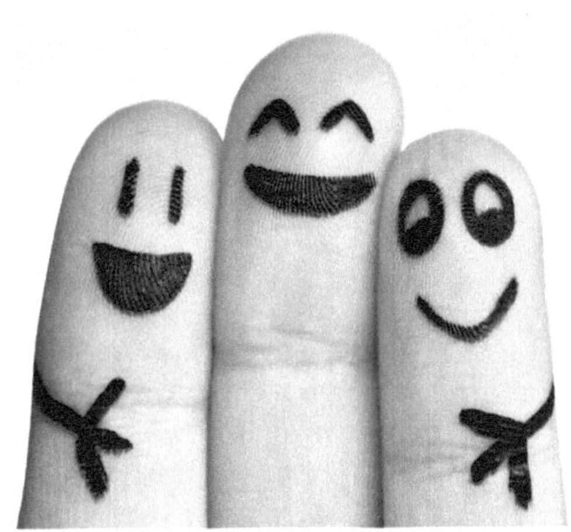

-   **Regulates your adrenal glands**

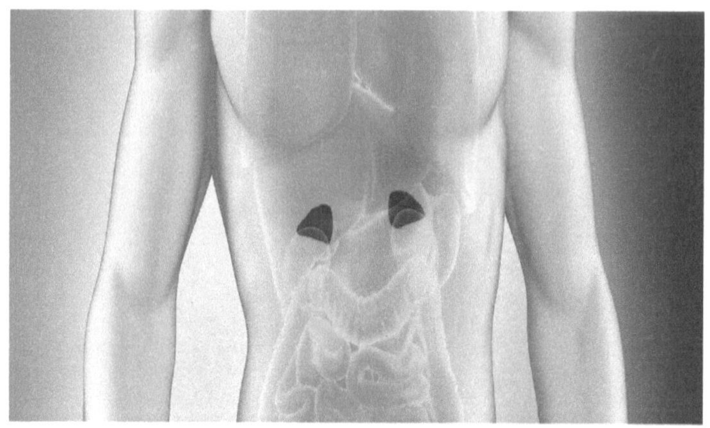

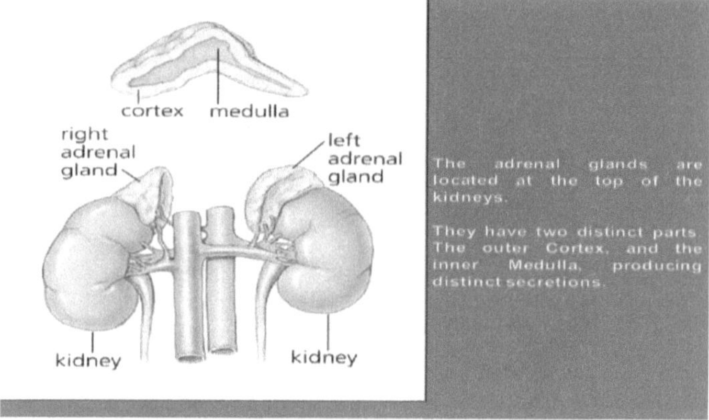

- **Drops your blood pressure**

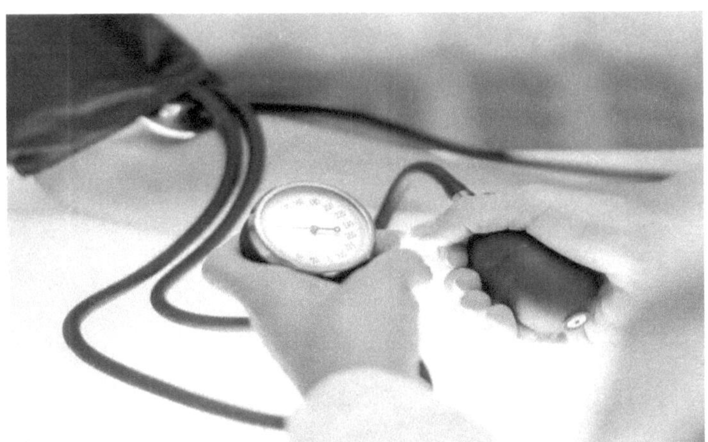

BLOOD PRESSURE CATEGORY	SYSTOLIC mm Hg (upper number)		DIASTOLIC mm Hg (lower number)
NORMAL	LESS THAN 120	and	LESS THAN 80
ELEVATED	120 – 129	and	LESS THAN 80
HIGH BLOOD PRESSURE (HYPERTENSION) STAGE 1	130 – 139	or	80 – 89
HIGH BLOOD PRESSURE (HYPERTENSION) STAGE 2	140 OR HIGHER	or	90 OR HIGHER
HYPERTENSIVE CRISIS (consult your doctor immediately)	HIGHER THAN 180	and/or	HIGHER THAN 120

- **Ups your heart rate**

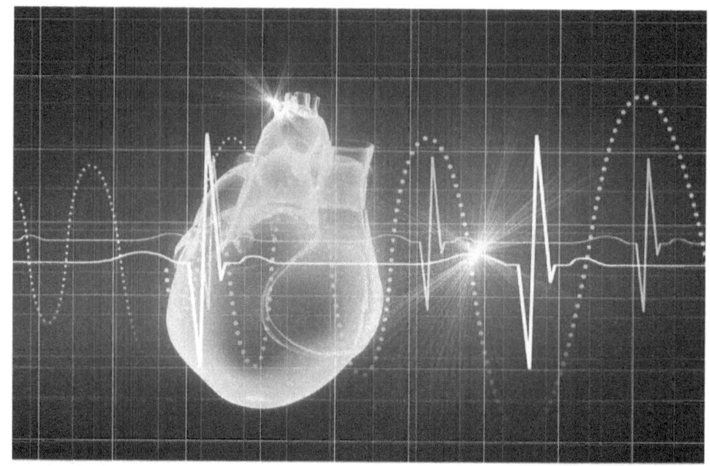

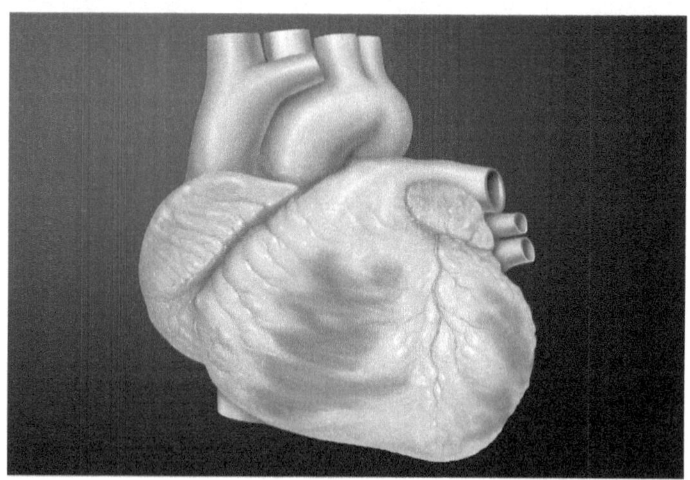

- **Drains your lymphs and boosts immunity**

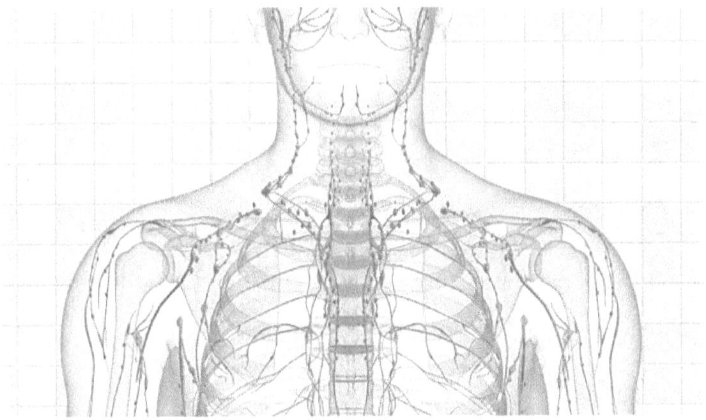

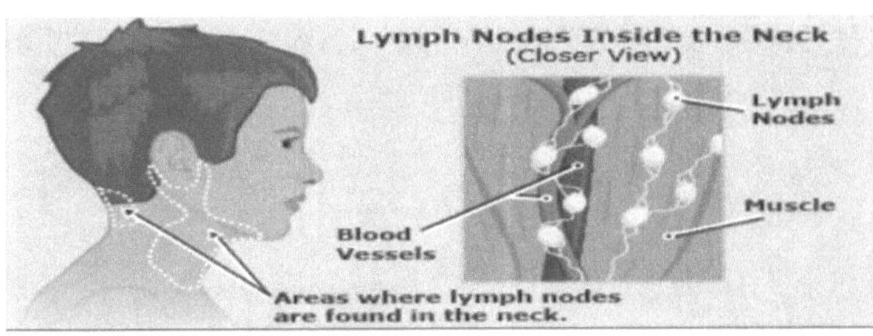

LYMPHADENITIS

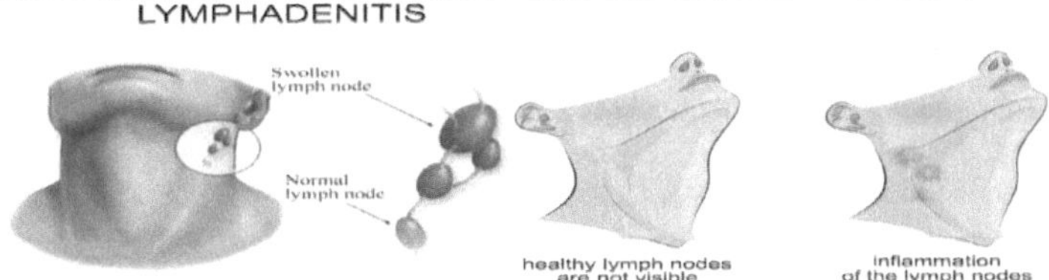

- **Increases your blood flow**

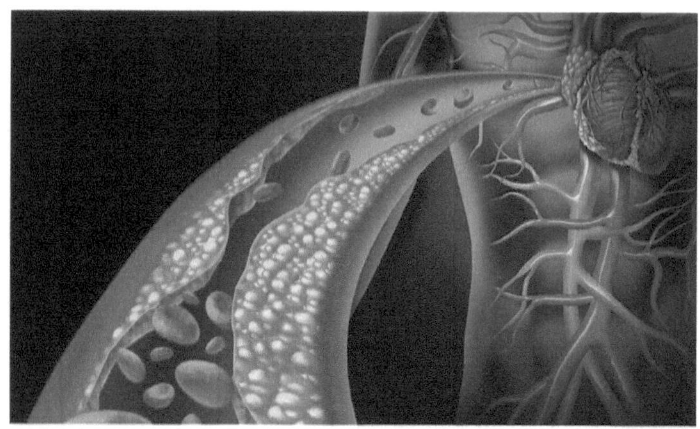

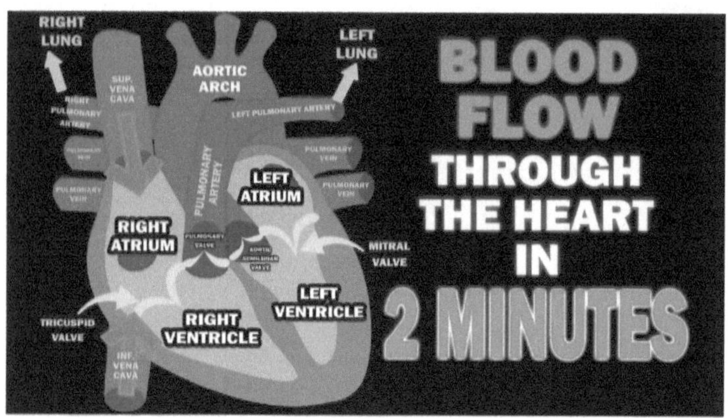

-   **Betters your bone health**

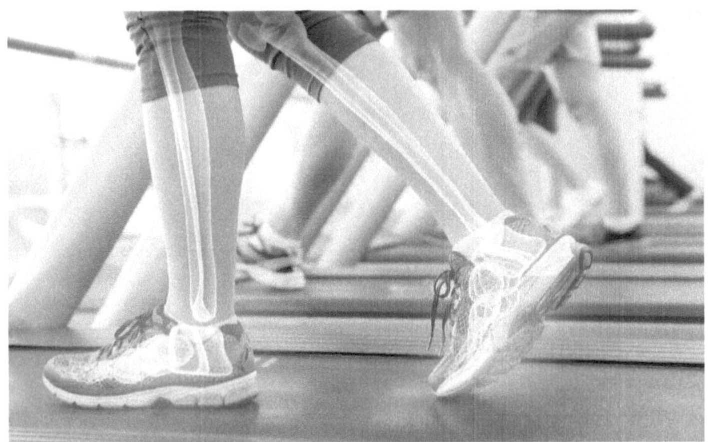

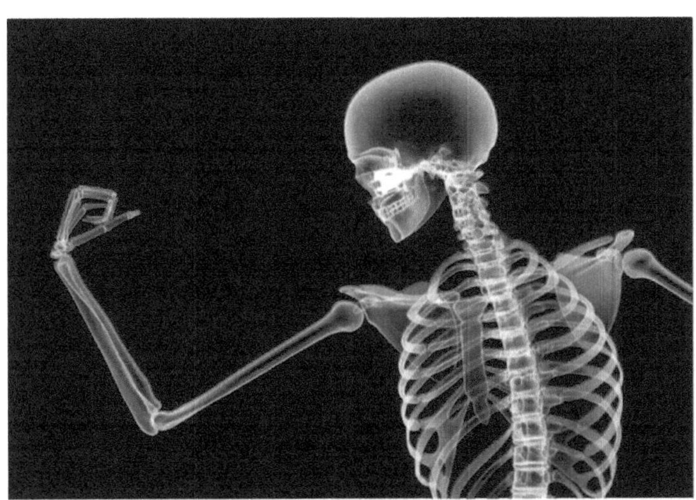

- **Protects your spine**

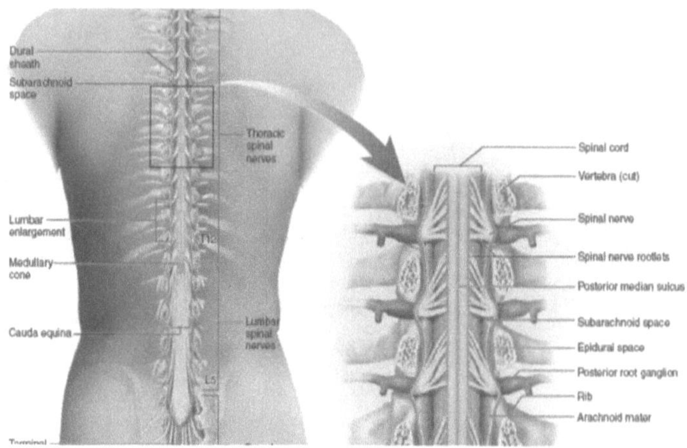

- **Prevents cartilage and joint breakdown**

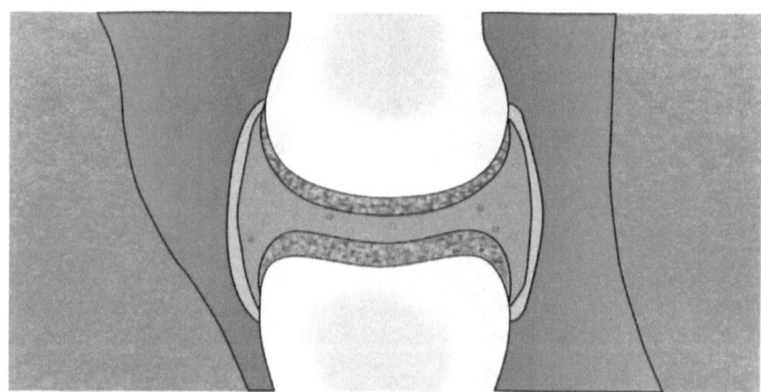

- **Perfects your posture**

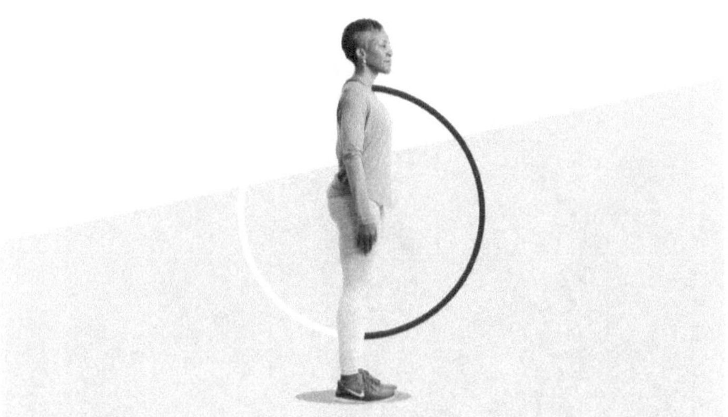

- **Builds muscle strength**

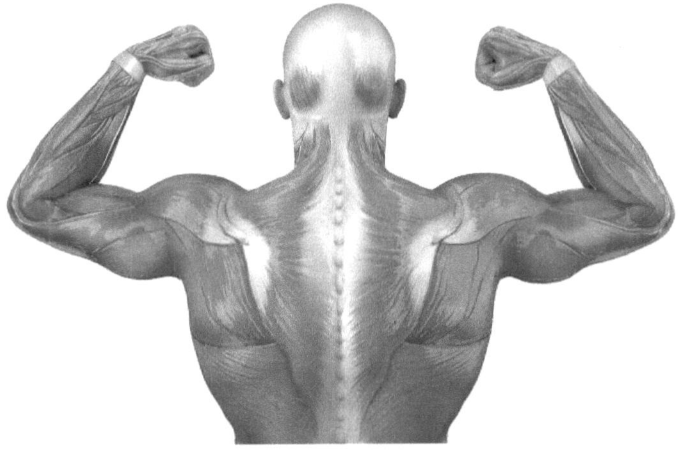

-    **Improves your flexibility**

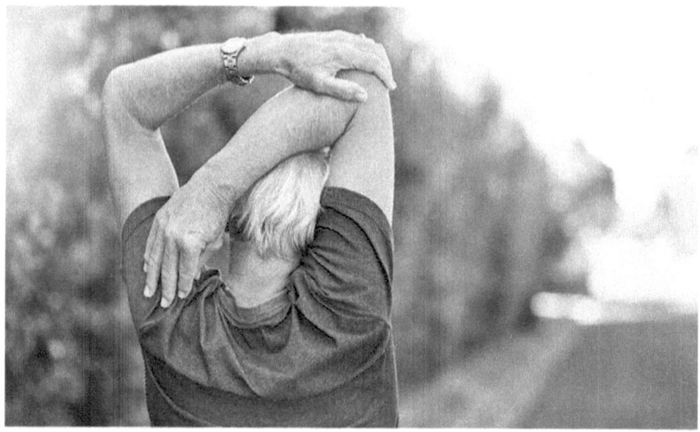

4. Types of Yoga

-   Acro yoga

AcroYoga is a dynamic physical practice that combines acrobatics, yoga and healing arts

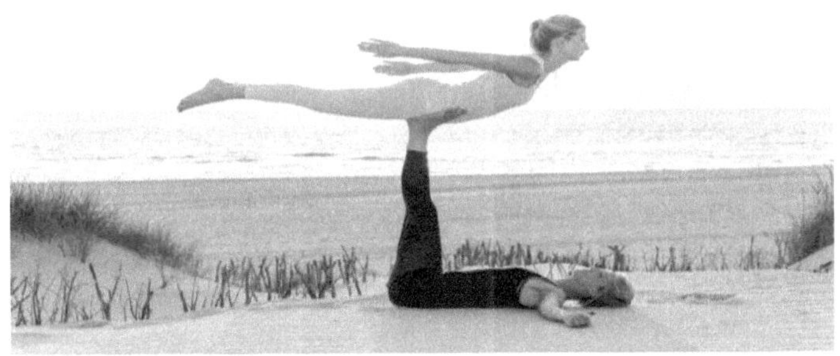

-   Aerial Yoga

Aerial yoga is a hybrid type of yoga developed in 2014 combining traditional yoga poses, Pilates, and dance with the use of a hammock

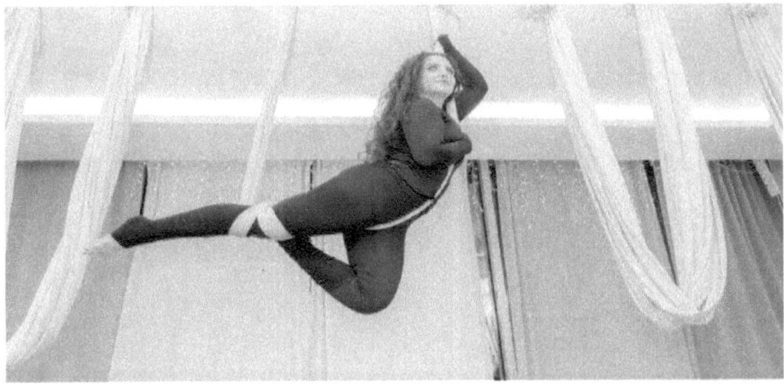

-   Prenatal Yoga

Prenatal yoga is a multifaceted approach to exercise that encourages stretching, mental centering and focused breathing

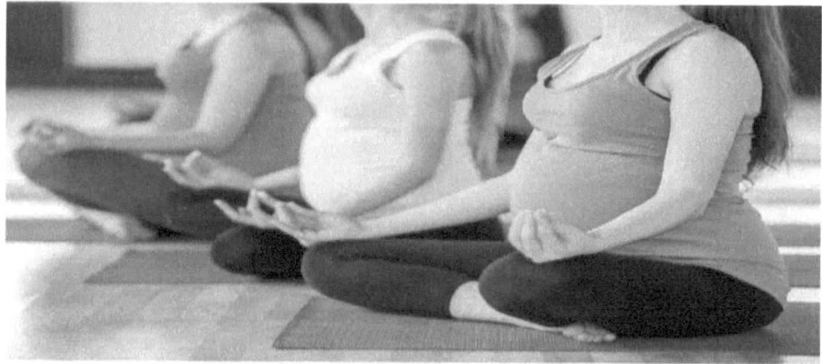

-   Restorative Yoga

Restorative yoga is simply that - restorative. It is the centering of your breath and body - aligning the physical and mental by practicing stillness

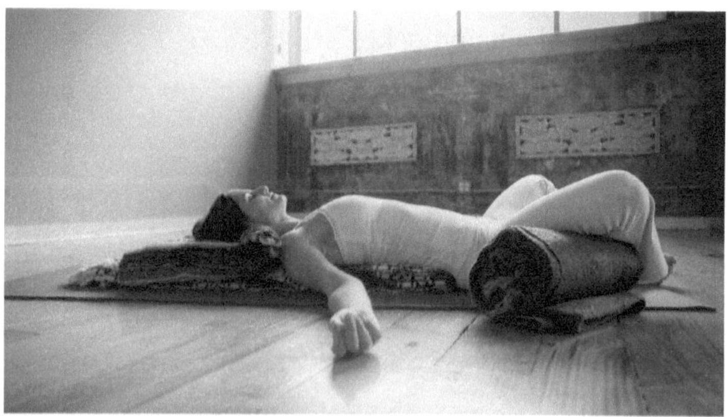

- Sivananda Yoga

Sivananda is one of the slower-paced styles of yoga that focuses more on meditation, breathing, and spirituality

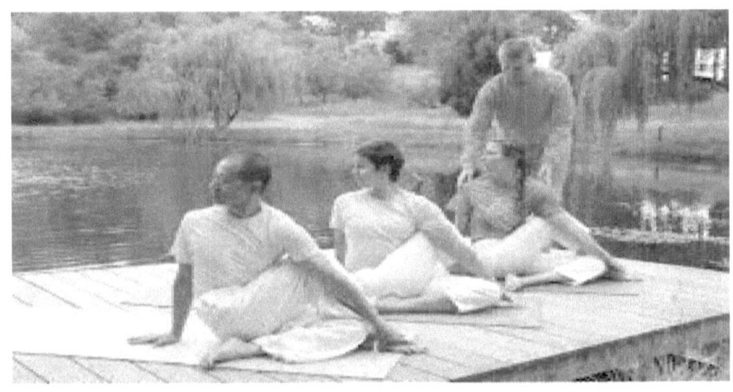

- Power Yoga

Power yoga is basically the lovechild of strength training and stretching. Here's a great total-body workout you can do with or without weights

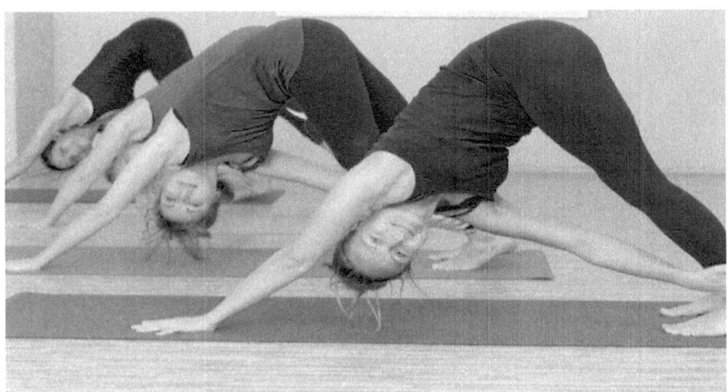

- **Bikram Yoga**

Bikram yoga is a type of yoga that involves a sequence of set poses and is usually done in a hot room at or above body temperature

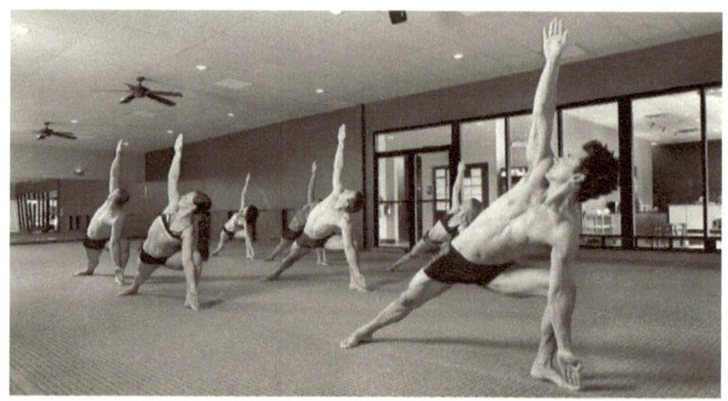

- **Iyengar Yoga**

Iyengar is a type of Hatha yoga where the focus in on alignment as well as the union of body, mind and soul

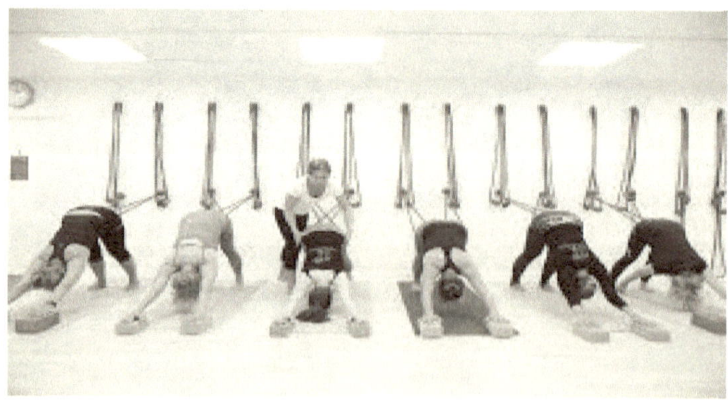

- **Yin Yoga**

Yin approach works to promote flexibility in areas often perceived as nonmalleable, especially the hips, pelvis, and lower spine

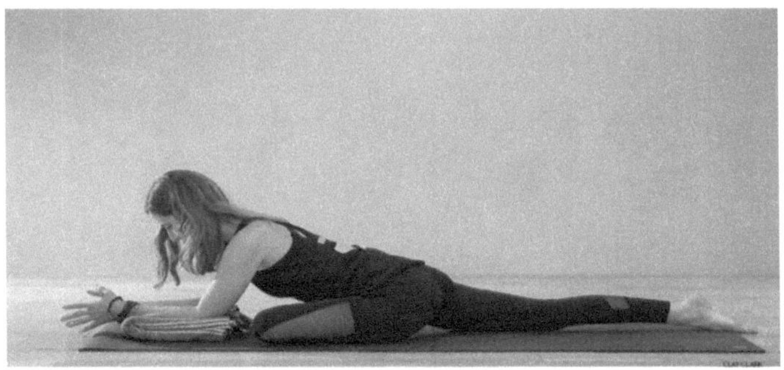

- **Ashtanga Yoga**

Ashtanga yoga is a system of yoga recorded by the sage Vamana Rishi in the Yoga Korunta, an ancient manuscript "said to contain lists of many different groupings of asanas, as well as highly original teachings on vinyasa, drishti, bandhas, mudras, and philosophy"

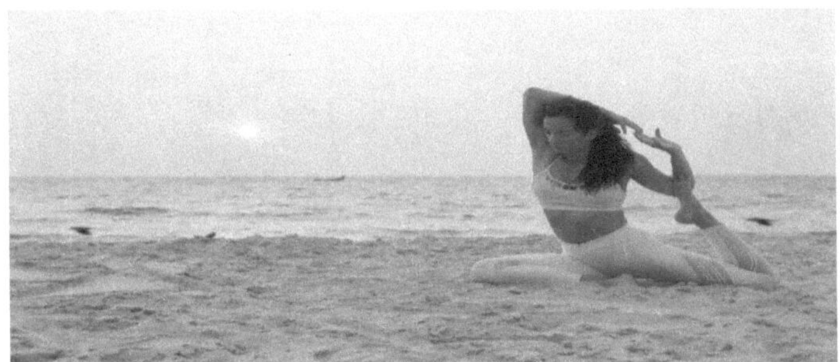

- Hatha Yoga

Hatha simply refers to the practice of physical yoga postures, meaning your Ashtanga, vinyasa, Iyengar and Power Yoga classes are all Hatha Yoga

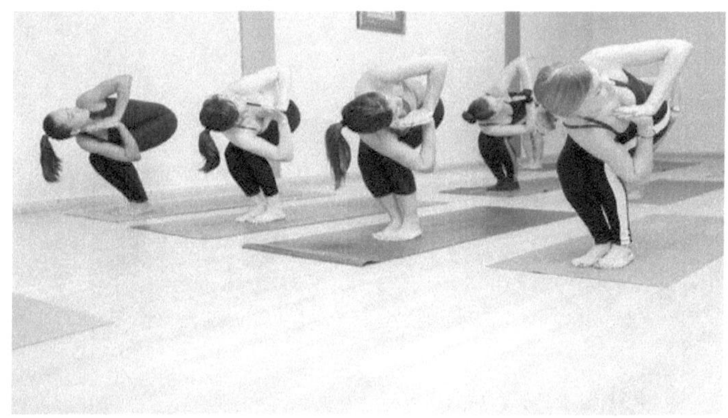

- Vinyasa Yoga

Vinyasa is a style of yoga characterized by stringing postures together so that you move from one to another, seamlessly, using breath

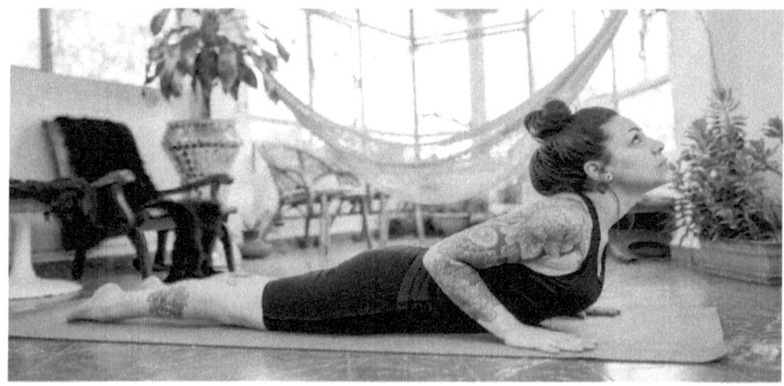

- **Kundalini Yoga**

Kundalini Yoga is little of both, but with an added emphasis on consciousness that activates energy centers throughout the body

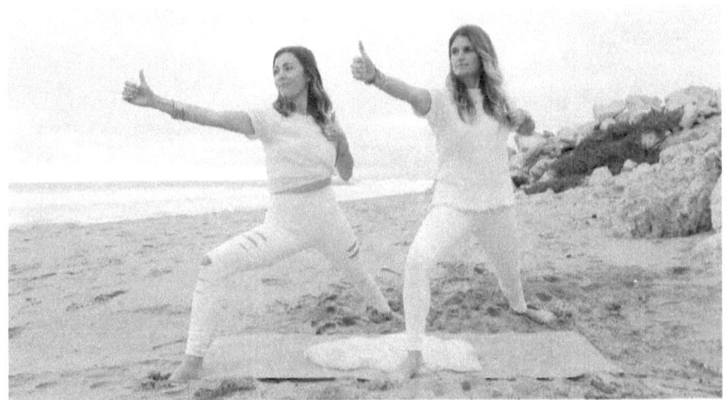

Thank you friend for getting our eBook.

If you have any question, please feel free to contact us.

Thank you